The Heat Protocol

Halt Covid-19 in 2hrs

Dr. Biswaroop Roy Chowdhury

DIAMOND BOOKS

India Office:
C/o India Book of Records
B-121, 2nd Floor, Greenfields,
Faridabad -120003 (Haryana),
India
Ph.: +91-9312286540

Malaysia Office:
C/o Bishwaroop International Healing & Research
PT 573, Lot 15077 Jalan Tuanku
Munawir,
70000 Negeri Sembilan, Malaysia
Tel: +6012-2116089

Vietnam Office:
C/o Vietnam Book of Records
148 Hong Ha Street
9 Award, Phu Nhuan District,
Ho Chi Minh City, Vietnam
- Hotline: (+84) 903710505

Switzerland Office:
C/o Nigel Kingsley
Kraftwerkstr. 95, ch-5465, Mellikon,
Switzerland
Tel: 0041 79 222 2323

FOLLOW ME

Facebook: https://www.facebook.com/drbrc.official/
Twitter: https://twitter.com/drbrcofficial
Bitchute: https://www.bitchute.com/channel/drbiswarooproychowdhury/
Instagram: https://www.instagram.com/dr.biswarooproychowdhury/
Telegram: https://t.me/drbiswarooproychowdhury
Email: biswaroop@biswaroop.com
Website: www.biswaroop.com
Video Channel: www.coronakaal.tv

Research : Rachna Sharma
NICE & Emergency Team: Kalpana Bourai, Pratiksha Vats, Shweta Jalhotra, Dr Namita Gupta, Dr Sangam Chopra, Sheetal Kanwar, Dr Iqra Shaikh
Copy Editor: Dr. Shubha P Wadhwa
Graphics Desinger: Shankar Singh Koranga

Published by
Diamond Pocket Books
X-30, Okhla Industrial Area, New Delhi-110020
Ph: 011-40712100 email: sales@dpb.in website: www.diamondbook.in

Dedication

Dedicated to all NICE/WISE experts, EPM Paramedics, Diabetes Educators & HIIMS Doctors/Nurses, who had faith in my research and helped me to spread DIP Diet/N.I.C.E Protocol & Postural Medicine to the masses.

Contents

Heat as Medicine

This book is based on the special training provided to N.I.C.E./ W.I.S.E. experts, EPM paramedics, Diabetes Educators and HIIMS Doctors/Nurses. To access the complete training video, go to **www.biswaroop.com/heatprotocol**

Heat as Medicine is a special training for everyone especially the N.I.C.E. experts (Network of Influenza Care), W.I.S.E. experts (Wellness and Inflammatory Syndrome Experts), students of Lincoln University, Shridhar University, EPM paramedics, doctors, staff and nurses of HIIMS hospital (Hospital and Institute of Integrated Medical Sciences) and Diabetes Educators from Indo-Vietnam Medical Board. Imagine you fall sick, how would you like yourself to be treated? I am sure your answer would be - through any method that is fastest, safest, cheapest and most importantly, evidence based or scientifically proven. What is that method? The first method that strikes a large majority of the people is Allopathy. What does the evidence reveal? All the major evidences I have collected are included in my book **"The Case Against IMA"** and by reading them, you would realize that Allopathy is nothing but an organized quackery. On the other hand, in the last two years, you have been acquainted with "food as medicine"- the three step Flu diet-the N.I.C.E. protocol. My book **"N.I.C.E. Way to Cure Covid-19"** was launched on 25 July, 2020 and with the help of this book, thousands of people could cure themselves of Flu/Covid-19. This method is scientifically proven and is the cheapest, safest, fastest and scientifically proven with zero mortality, no side effects and within three days a person can get rid of the Flu (it might take seven days for about 5% people and may be 10 days for 1% people). In contrast to this, if we consider the conventional WHO protocol, there are 12% chances that a person won't return from the hospital; he may die. If he comes back (88% chances), he carries along a number of other diseases such as kidney failure, Diabetes, Arthritis etc. He does not return back to normalcy.

Whenever you choose a particular method of treatment, question yourself if this method is safest, fastest, cheapest and most importantly, evidence based. The three step Flu diet qualifies all these conditions. You learnt through DIP diet that people who had been taking medication for Diabetes, blood pressure etc. for a long time (10, 20, 30 years or more) could get rid of them in a few days (5-7-10 days). Can we call it the fastest method? Of course, yes. Can we call Allopathy as the fastest method? No, Not at all. It is quite clear that by consuming allopathic medicines, you always remain sick. One thing is for sure that your illness keeps increasing. You have seen how lakhs of people cured themselves in just a few days through DIP diet which we call "food as medicine".

You also noticed that through postural medicine, several hundred people who were on dialysis and were recommended kidney transplant, could get rid of medicines within a few days; some people could get rid of dialysis from the first day itself. Surely, gravity as medicine i.e. postural medicine is the safest, fastest and cheapest method. Gravitational force cannot be purchased from a shop; it is freely available around us.

Next is heat as medicine. Heat is also easily available in nature-in the form of sunlight, fire etc. Heat can help cure Flu in the safest, fastest and cheapest manner and it is scientifically proven. Flu/Covid 19/ Influenza like Illness/Omicron/NeoCov or any other respiratory virus can be flushed out from our body by using heat as medicine. By using heat as medicine, you will have to spend as little as two hours.

As soon as the first symptom of Flu appears in a person-be it cough, cold, bodyache, weakness or high temperature, he should follow this revolutionary method that would cure him in the time till the ambulance arrives-that is, within a span of half an hour to two hours. Through this training, I hand over my research to you; now it is your responsibility to apply this research/ training on yourself or your friends, if suffering from a Flu.

The occurrence of Flu is not bad; every person catches Flu once or twice in a year. Flu has been given a trendy name these days. What is known as Omicron today, was called Delta a few days back. So don't get confused with the names. The moment the first symptom of Flu appears, use heat as medicine. You will adopt this three step heat protocol about which we will learn here. You yourself will realize that most of the patients get cured within a span of two hours.

To begin with the training, let us first understand what is Flu or respiratory disease? Actually it is called Influenza Like Illness (ILI). Rhino virus, common cold virus, Corona virus, novel corona virus or any other variants, which enter the body through nose and mouth, are called respiratory viruses. However powerful they may be, they die through certain methods. Most importantly, you need to understand that all these respiratory viruses have the tendency to make variants. That is why they are called viruses. Every year, most of us suffer from Flu (ILI) and soon recover. The recovery itself indicates that your body has developed the antibodies towards that virus and those antibodies remove that virus from the body. Have you ever wondered that when antibodies are developed in the body, why do we get fever again? This is because the virus, which was responsible for your fever and common cold, has mutated so the antibodies developed earlier cannot tackle the new variant and new antibodies need to be developed altogether. This is the reason that right from our childhood we get infected with viruses thousands of times. You need to understand that the antibodies developed by our body are not permanent because next time when the virus attacks, it would have already mutated. Mutation is its tendency and that is why you get common cold so often. If it did not mutate, we would have suffered from Flu and common cold just once in our entire lives. Thus, the mutation of virus is something very common and hence we suffer from Flu and common cold quite often. The more you are attacked by viruses, the more you tend to strengthen your immunity. If this does not occur, your immunity will not exert itself. It is the same thing as if you don't exercise your muscles, they would become weak. This is the reason so many people go to the Gym to exercise their muscles. The same is the case with our immunity. If it is not used, it will become weak. When you get Flu or common cold, the immunity gets an opportunity to rehearse itself. That is why having Flu or ILI or Omicron is not strange or bad; nor can anyone escape it. Virus is not our enemy; it is a synchronization of humans and viruses. We are all surrounded by viruses but do we always fall sick? No, because a harmony exists between the human beings and the viruses.

Imagine the society /colony where you reside. There exists a harmony between you and the dogs present there. The society/colony belongs to those dogs also. You don't oblige them by giving them some food; they also play a significant role in your lives. They shoo away the insects and other harmful animals from entering your colony. So they are providing you several kinds of protection. In this way, a balance in nature is maintained.

Now, imagine a situation when you lose sight in the night time and unintentionally step up on the tail of the dog. What will happen? The dog, which normally doesn't bite you, will now bite you. That doesn't mean that dogs are bad or they should not stay in the colony. If the dog has bitten you, it is more of your fault rather than the dog's. You broke the rule. You hurt the dog unintentionally. What is to be corrected is your eyesight; you don't have to shoo the dog away. If you don't pay attention to your eyesight and kick the dog away, you might harm some other dog later (because of your poor eyesight) and it too would bite you. If you think you will kill all the dogs, it is not correct. They too have a role to play-to protect you from thieves, snakes, rats, cats and other insects thereby maintaining a balance in nature. If the dogs are killed, there would be plenty of snakes, rats, cats and other insects and an imbalance would be created in nature.

There may be a situation where the dog has gone mad. In this case, it would bite not only you but others till you remove the dog from your locality.

The same relation is shared by the respiratory viruses and human beings. The respiratory tract is the normal residence of these viruses. If you get yourself checked now, you would find several viruses-rhino virus, novel corona virus, Omicron and others present in your nose. They maintain the balance. They attack you when your immunity is weakened. It is not the virus to be blamed but you yourself are at fault since you have weakened your immunity through your actions or habits. Here you cannot kill all the viruses. Therefore, it is important to strengthen your immunity. There may be a situation when the number of viruses increase in your body; the balance is not maintained so in such a case, you need to reduce the number of viruses by destroying them.

You might have noticed during the so called first wave and second wave of Corona, some people returned from the hospital after a week or a month while others didn't return at all. On the one hand, you saw that some people who went to the hospital were on treatment for months together and several people died also and on the other hand, this book claims that a person can recover from Flu/Covid 19 in just two hours. Isn't it contradictory? Whenever you kill a virus or for that matter any creature, the time to kill depends upon the method being used.

Any respiratory virus especially SARSCoV-2, which has been publicized so much these days (there is no pandemic; it's all propaganda), if kept at 20^0C, will survive for 28 days. If the temperature is increased to 40^0C, the virus will die in less than 24 hours.

Heat As Medicine

SARSCoV-2 survives for
28 days at 20°C
Less than 24 hours at 40°C

Riddell, S., Goldie, S., Hill, A. et al. The effect of temperature on persistence of SARS-CoV-2 on common surfaces. Virol J 17, 145 (2020).

Here, heat is the medicine. The survival of the virus depends upon the temperature. When the patients used to go to the hospital or even when they go today with the Flu symptoms, the hospital is sometimes air-conditioned and when they put on the oxygen cylinder, a cold wave is formed. As a result, the Flu turns into Pneumonia. The steroids or the Paracetamol that are administered to the patients do not kill the virus. Virus is a non-living thing but it behaves like a living thing inside the living creature (say human). What we can do is to deactivate the virus so that it doesn't behave like a living thing and does not multiply and spread to the entire body. How can that be done? By using heat as medicine. When we heat the virus at 60^{0}C for 30 minutes, it becomes inactive and gets destroyed. If the temperature is increased further, it gets destroyed in 15 minutes; and at 80^{0}C, the virus is destroyed in one minute.

Heat As Medicine

Corona virus becomes inactive

60°C for 30 min

65°C for 15 min

80°C for 1 min

Kampf G, Voss A, Scheithauer S. Inactivation of coronaviruses by heat. J Hosp Infect. 2020; 105(2):348-349. doi:10.1016/j.jhin.2020.03.025

As soon as you provide heat to the virus especially Corona virus, the spike protein that binds the virus to the body, gets destroyed. The structure of the protein is denatured; it can neither replicate nor latch itself with the cells of the body. How can this happen? With heat. Yes, of course with heat. You might be surprised that on the one hand, a person goes to the hospital to get himself treated for Flu either does not return or if he returns alive, it may be after a week or a month and on the other hand, is the treatment in just two hours. Yes, this is true. It depends upon the method used to kill the virus. Let me question you. If we have to kill a person, how long will it take? It depends on the kind of weapon used for killing purpose. Remember, human beings and viruses are not immortal. If a human being is free from diseases, even then he would die. 100 years is the normal life span of a human being. If he is deprived of food, then he will die within three to four weeks. In the absence of water, he would die in 3-4 days. If he is deprived of oxygen, he will lose his life within 3-4 minutes and if he is beheaded, he will die in 4-30 seconds (not immediately).

Killing Human		Killing Virus	
100 years	Normal Lifespan	Paracetamol Antibiotics Steroids	Full Lifespan
3-4 weeks	No food	60°C	30 min
3-4 days	No water	65°C	15 min
3-4 min	No Oxygen	80°C	1 min
4-30 sec	Beheaded	100°C	Few seconds

Similar is the case with viruses. The destruction of virus depends upon the method adopted. If you ask the people who got themselves treated for Flu at the hospitals, which strategy was used to kill the virus, they would tell you that they were given Paracetamol, steroids and antibiotics. Do you think Paracetamol can kill the vius? No, not at all. It rather saves the virus from destruction. Paracetamol reduces the temperature of your body; so as heat reduces, the growth of virus aggravates. Similarly, steroids and antibiotics weaken the immunity. All these medicines create a healthy environment for the spread of the virus, which ultimately destroys the entire body. Unfortunately, the medication provided in the hospitals is targeted at the destruction of human beings not the virus. Rather, a suitable environment is set up for the virus to flourish. For evidence, you may refer to my book **"Delta 72"**, which is freely available on my website **www.biswaroop.com/delta72.**

It is often noticed that despite this medication for Flu, some people are saved. It is purely because of their good luck or strong immunity. Even through, they are recover from Flu they suffer from other diseases throughout their lives. Remember, the virus will continue to exist in the body throughout his life and we attribute White fungus, Black fungus etc. to Corona; actually they are the result of medication provided in the hospital. The important part is despite being aware of all this, nobody protests against these medicines. There is no evidence to prove that by giving Paracetamol to the patient, virus is killed whereas there are ample evidences to prove it otherwise. The best way to kill the virus is by using heat. If the virus Is kept at 60^{0}C, it gets killed in 30 minutes; at 65^{0}C, virus gets destroyed in 15 minutes; at 80^{0}C, it gets killed in one minute and at 100^{0}C, it gets destroyed in a few seconds. Thus it depends on the weapon used to kill- be it a human being or a virus. Therefore, when you have Flu, it may take a week to recover; it actually depends on what action are you taking during that time. If you apply the strategy of medication, it will take a very very long time to recover since you are creating suitable conditions for the growth of the virus.

Do you know that when a vaccine is made against a particular virus, the virus is deactivated and introduced in the vaccine. Now, how is the virus deactivated by the manufacturing companies? Does it use Paracetamol, steroids or antibiotics to deactivate the virus? No, not at all. The company heats the virus in order to deactivate it and puts it into the vaccine.

In vaccine manufacturing, virus is deactivated by heating the virus
Darnell ME, Subbarao K, Feinstone SM, Taylor DR. Inactivation of the coronavirus that induces severe acute respiratory syndrome, SARS-CoV. J Virol Methods. 2004; 121(1):85-91. doi:10.1016/j.jviromet. 2004.06.006

This is how a vaccine is made. The strategy that is used in the making of a vaccine, the very same strategy is to be used in destroying the virus in the body.

Here is the model to get rid of the virus.

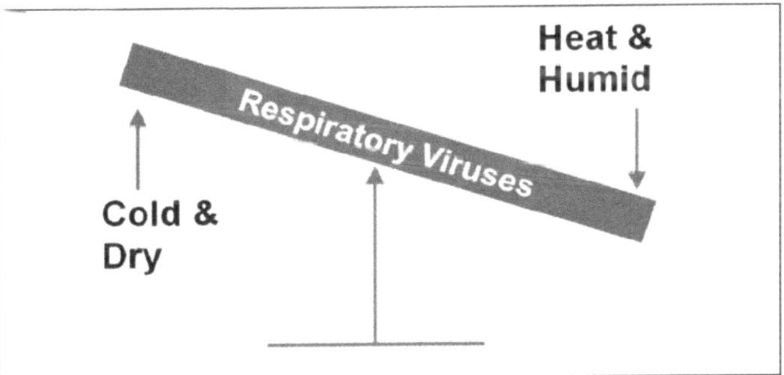

Kudo E, Song E, Yockey LJ, et al.: Low ambient humidity impairs barrier function and innate resistance against influenza infection. Proc Natl Acad Sci U S A. 2019; 116(22): 10905–10910.

Any respiratory virus flourishes in cold and dry conditions and gets destroyed in hot and humid conditions. Since our aim is to destroy the virus, we need to somehow provide it heat. How rapidly will it be destroyed will depend on the amount and speed of heat provided to the virus. This is simple science/principle which has already been proved.

BARRIERS FOR VIRUS

As stated earlier, respiratory virus travels to our body through nose and mouth. In fact, it already exists in our nose. However, there are barriers in our respiratory tract especially in the nose which ensure that this virus may not harm us.

Barrier for Virus

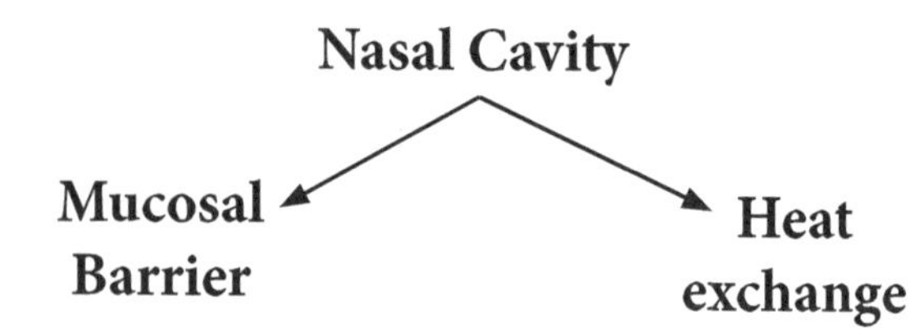

Soni B, Nayak AK: Effect of inspiration cycle and ventilation rate on heat exchange in human respiratory airways.
- J Therm Biol. 2019; 84: 357–367
Fahy JV, Dickey BF: Airway mucus function and dysfunction.
- N Engl J Med. 2010; 363(23): 2233–2247

There are two barriers- one is mucosal barrier i.e. a semi-liquid layer which stops the viruses from entering inside the body. The second one is heat exchange which does not allow the virus to spread.

HEAVEN FOR VIRUS

It is often seen that in the winter season, we do not get proper sunlight. This condition becomes the heaven for the virus. In that case, our nose is the coldest part of our body which is very conducive to the growth of viruses. That means, the more we are away from the sunlight, the more are the chances of virus spreading in our body.

Heaven for Virus

Winter → Restricted Sunlight

→ Dry Air

↓

Nasal cavity becomes coldest part of the body

Soni B, Nayak AK: Effect of inspiration cycle and ventilation rate on heat exchange in human respiratory airways.
- J Therm Biol. 2019; 84: 357–367
Fahy JV, Dickey BF: Airway mucus function and dysfunction.
- N Engl J Med. 2010; 363(23): 2233–2247

What is the solution? When the first symptom of Flu occurs, you should immediately take the following measures. You should apply heat to the body so that the virus is flushed out immediately. Heat helps in direct inhibition of pathogens; as a result viruses do not multiply and are flushed out. Indirectly, when heat is applied to the body, it activates our immunity. Heat also reduces inflammatory responses and prevents tissue damage. In this way, the spread of viruses is restricted.

Heat applied to the body

- **Direct inhibition of pathogen**
- **Stimulation of innate & adaptive arm of immune system.**
- **Reduce inflammatory response**
- **Prevents tissue damage**

Evans SS, Repasky EA, Fisher DT: Fever and the thermal regulation of immunity: the immune system feels the heat.
- Nat Rev Immunol. 2015; 15(6): 335–349

We must also understand that the application of heat creates a kind of artificial fever. Fever is not the cause of any infection. In fact, when there is some pathological infection in our body, fever acts as a weapon to fight against that infection. When we provide heat to

Heat stress applied on body to mimic fever thus supporting and activating immune system, the second line of defense.

Schieber AMP, Ayres JS: Thermoregulation as a disease tolerance defense strategy.
-Pathog Dis. 2016; 74(9); pii: ftw106

Mace TA, Zhong L, Kilpatrick C, et al.: Differentiation of CD8+ T cells into effector cells is enhanced by physiological range hyperthermia.
- J Leukoc Biol. 2011; 90(5): 951–962

our body, an artificial fever is generated, which helps in activating our immunity and strengthens the defence system to fight against viruses.

STAGES OF DEFENCE MECHANISM

There are two stages of the defence mechanism:

STAGE 1

Direct application of heat to upper airways, at the first sign of infection inhibits virus replication. With the first symptom of cold, cough, fever, bodyache or weakness, if you give heat to the respiratory area i.e. on mouth and nose, you would start feeling better.

Defense – Stage 1
Direct application of heat to upper airways, at the first sign of infection inhibits virus replication.
Conti C, De Marco A, Mastromarino P, et al.: Antiviral effect of hyperthermic treatment in rhinovirus infection. *- Antimicrob Agents Chemother. 1999; 43(4): 822–829*

STAGE 2

Whenever heat is provided to the body, it starts making the blood alkaline, which helps in boosting the immunity thus preventing the spread of virus. The question is how will we provide heat? Skin is the barrier. It is, in fact, the medium which helps heat to enter into our body.

Defense – Stage 2

Heat stress (on body) alters blood pH, creating alkaline condition – favourable condition for immune system.

Tsuji B, Hayashi K, Kondo N, et al.: Characteristics of hyperthermia-induced hyperventilation in humans. -Temperature (Austin). 2016; 3(1): 146–160

Skin can be considered as the third kidney. Skin performs the same functions as our kidneys. Here are a few facts about skin in comparison to the kidneys.

1. Skin has 22% blood supply, which is the same as our kidneys.
2. Skin eliminates approximately 12 litres of water/fluid from the body. On the other hand, kidneys eliminate approximately 10 litres.
3. Skin excretes various unwanted or excess chemicals like sodium, potassium, urea, creatinine, calcium, phosphorous, glucose drug substance and heavy metals from our body in the form of sweat in the same way as excretion of chemicals is done during the urination process. So sweating is due to skin and urination is due to kidneys. Those people in whom the urine output is nil, their urine can be excreted through the skin by heating the body. Thus

skin is one such organ through which you can unlock any organ in the body.

Skin – The Third Kidney

- **Blood supply – 22% of cardiac output**
- **Ability to eliminate – 12 L liquid**
- **Skin excretes sodium, potassium, urea, creatinine, calcium, phosphorous, glucose, drug substance and heavy metals.**

Benet L. Pharmacokinetics: The dynamics of drug absorption, distribution and elimination. The Pharmacological Basis of Therapeutics. MacMillan, New York 1996:22

KEY TO ACTIVATE SKIN

In order to activate the skin, there should be an increase in body temperature and increase in sweat. If the temperature of the skin is increased, the sweating of the body too would increase. How to increase the temperature of the skin?

Key to activate skin

Rise in temperature & rise in sweat (10°C rise in temperature triples sweating)

Diamandopoulos AA, Goudas PC. Substitution of renal function through skin catharsis: evidence from the classical period to the Middle Ages. Kidney Int. 2001 Apr; 59(4):1580-9

To control the virus within 1 to 2 hours of getting the first symptom of Flu, the following therapies should be taken.

1. LOWER LEG HOT WATER IMMERSION

Lower Leg Hot Water immersion therapy helps in curing the infection. In this therapy, the lower part of legs are dipped in hot water. This increases the immune response of the body because heat is being provided to the body through the legs.

Lower Leg Hot Water Immersion

- **Improves immune response**
- **Improves blood circulation**
- **Counteracting infection**
- **Effective in reducing body temperature**

Diamandopoulos AA, Goudas PC. Substitution of renal function through skin catharsis: evidence from the classical period to the Middle Ages. Kidney Int. 2001 Apr; 59(4):1580-9

This also increases the blood circulation. It is medically proven that this therapy is also effective in reducing the body temperature. If a person is suffering from fever, by following the Lower Leg Hot Water Immersion therapy, fever can be reduced faster than by taking Paracetamol tablets.

Warm Water v/s Paracetamol

Rate of reduction of body temperature is faster in warm water therapy in first 30 min.

Aksoylar S, Akşit S, Cağlayan S, Yaprak I, Bakiler R, Cetin F. Evaluation of sponging and antipyretic medication to reduce body temperature in febrile children. Acta Paediatr Jpn. 1997 Apr; 39(2):215-7.

It is also observed that if you take Paracetamol, the fever again increases because medicine does not kill the virus; it rather deactivates the ability of the brain to increase the body temperature. On the other hand, Lower Leg Hot Water Immersion therapy activates the immunity of the body and helps in killing the virus. Hence, it's a reference-based technique. Thus, we can say it is the fastest, safest, cheapest and evidence based method of curing an ailment.

2. NASAL HYPER THERMIA

Similarly, nasal hyperthermia also gives immediate relief from viral infection. That means, if heat is provided to the body through the nose and the mouth along with Lower Leg Hot Water Immersion, it provides quick relief.

Nasal hyperthermia can give immediate relief from symptom.

Dyrrell D, Barrow I, Arthur J. Local hyperthermia benefits natural and experimental common colds. BMJ. 1989 May 13; 298(6683):1280-3. doi: 10.1136/bmj.298.6683.1280. Erratum in: BMJ 1989 Sep 2; 299(6699):600

To get comfort, feel energized and recover from Flu, follow the three step heat protocol.

STEP 1

When you observe the first sign of Flu such as cold, cough, fever or fatigue, you should take Lower Leg Hot Water Immersion (LLHWI) therapy i.e. take hot water (approx. 42 degrees to 43 degrees) in a bucket.

With 1st sign of Flu / 1st 30 min

STEP-I

Lower leg hot water immersion (42°C to 43°C)

With lavender oil

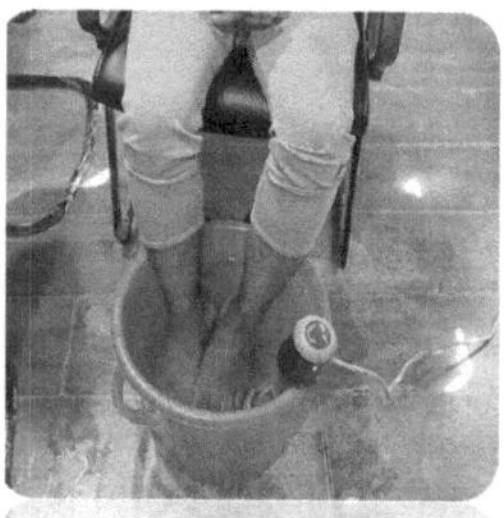

Babar Ali et al. Essential oils used in aromatherapy, A systemic review: July 2015 Asian Pacific Journal of Tropical Biomedicine 5(8):589-598

3 Step Heat Protocol

Add one tablespoon of Lavender oil in it. Dip your legs in the bucket. The aroma of Lavender oil de-stresses the patient and hot water cures the Flu effect. This therapy should be performed for about 30 minutes and while the legs are placed inside the bucket, the temperature of water should be maintained between 42-43 degrees. To maintain the temperature, keep another bucket full of water having temperature more than 50^{0}C; remove two mugs of water from the bucket in which the legs are dipped and add two mugs of water from the other bucket. If you repeat the process after every 5 minutes, it will ensure that the temperature of water is maintained to 42-43 degrees throughtout the duration of the first step. To make the LLHWI therapy more effective, you can put a blanket on the patient.

If the patient is too weak to sit down (since this therapy is best done while sitting), make him lie down and dip both his feet in hot water bucket as shown in the picture. In this case, the patient may forgo step 2 and step 3.

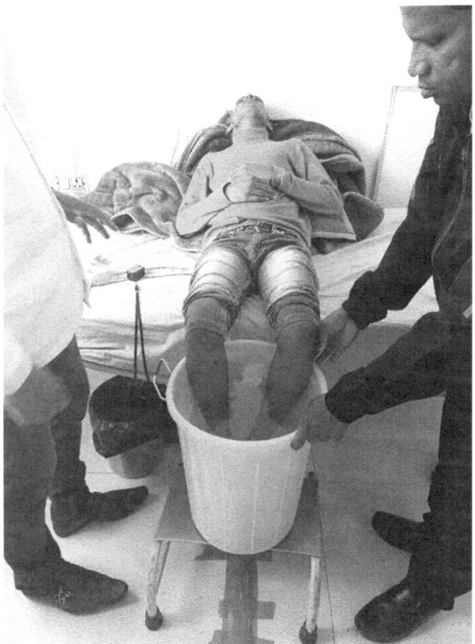

STEP 2

Take 500 ml hot water (whose temperature is approx. > 80°C). Squeeze one lemon (juice) in it. Start sipping it slowly. In this manner, we are providing heat and humidity through the nose and mouth, which helps in destroying the virus in its early stage.

With 1st sign of Flu / 1st 30 min

STEP-II

Sipping very-very hot water(>80°C) about 500 ml with lemon juice drops

3 Step Heat Protocol

STEP 3

The third step is nasal irrigation commonly known as Jal neti (one of the famous techniques mentioned in Ayurveda).

Take 200 ml hot water (approx. 40°C - 42°C). Add one spoon of salt in it and perform Jal neti as described in the Ayurveda. This procedure needs expertise.

With 1st sign of Flu / 1st 30 min

STEP-III

Nasal irrigation (Jal neti)(40°C to 42°C) about 200 ml with salt (one spoon)

3 Step Heat Protocol

To perform it in a simple manner, take a squeezy bottle (like tomato sause plastic bottle) and perform Jal neti for around 2-3 minutes. This step can also be done simultaneously with the first step.

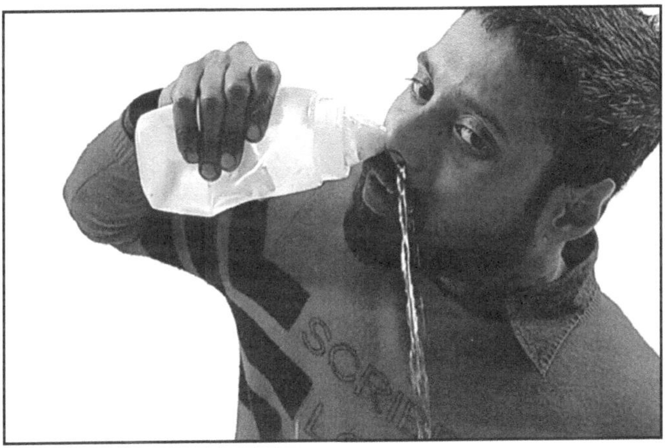

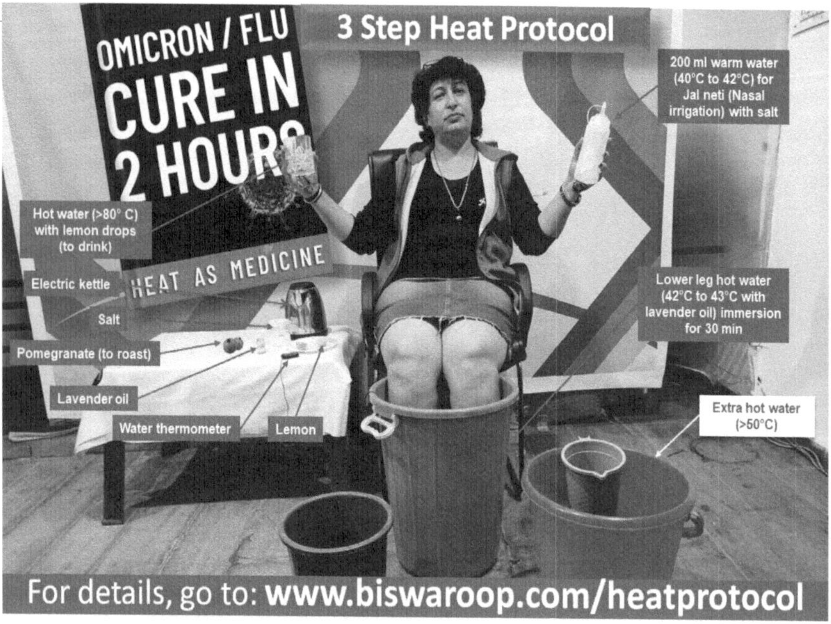
OMICRON / FLU
CURE IN
2 HOURS
3 Step Heat Protocol
200 ml warm water (40°C to 42°C) for Jal neti (Nasal irrigation) with salt
Hot water (>80° C) with lemon drops (to drink)
HEAT AS MEDICINE
Electric kettle
Salt
Pomegranate (to roast)
Lavender oil
Water thermometer
Lemon
Lower leg hot water (42°C to 43°C with lavender oil) immersion for 30 min
Extra hot water (>50°C)
For details, go to: www.biswaroop.com/heatprotocol

It is advised that by repeating the above three steps 2-3 times would provide relief from Flu. The three step heat protocol is depicted in brief:

3 Step Heat Protocol – 30 min	
Step I	→ LL HWI (Lavender oil)
Step II	→ Sipping very hot water (500 ml + Lemon)
Step III	Jal neti (200 ml water + salt)

It is also suggested that even after getting well, follow the three step Flu diet for 3 days.

Prevention

Repeat the 3 Step Heat Protocol 2-3 times the same day

+

Follow 3 Step Flu Diet

Read N.I.C.E way to Cure COVID-19 →

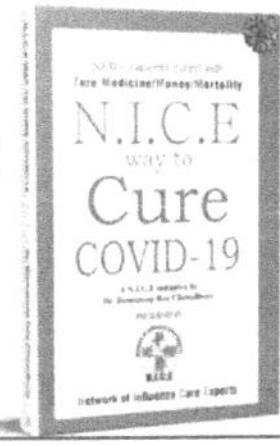

Apart from this, if a person is suffering from Whooping Cough, what to do? Take some Pomegranate seeds. For every 10 kg body weight, one spoon of Pomegranate seeds is required. For example, a person weighing 70 kg needs to have seven spoons of roasted Pomegranate seeds. Roast the seeds for 4- 5 minutes and chew them well while they are still hot. It would immediately relieve him of Whooping Cough.

Whooping Cough

Roast Pomegranate seeds for 4 to 5 minutes

+

Eat while they're hot

Heat As Medicine

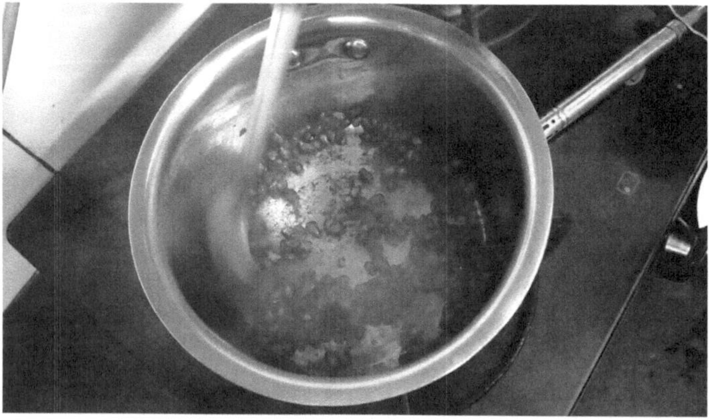

In a nutshell, we have learnt that by following the above steps, how a virus can be controlled/destroyed in its very first stage.

Moving on to the lifestyle diseases such as Pneumonia, Asthma, Tuberculosis, the person should apply the three step heat protocol

Treatment of respiratory illnesses (pneumonia, tuberculosis, asthma)

↓

3 Step Heat Protocol + DIP Diet (minus plate 2 in lunch)

↓

For one to 3 months

along with DIP diet. By doing so, one can get rid of the above diseases in one to three months.

For more details, you can go through the Training Manual, which is available on our website **www.biswaroop.com/heatprotocol**

To read, go to

www.biswaroop.com/heatprotocol

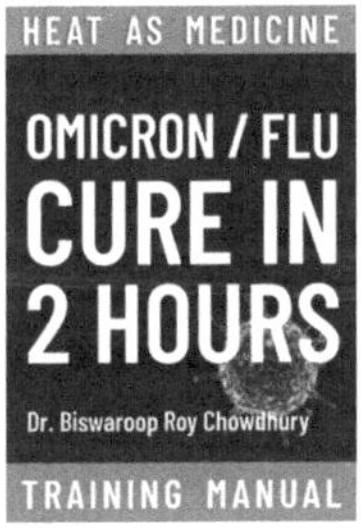

If you are convinced with the above therapies, do share more and more with your family and friends in order to provide maximum benefit to your near and dear ones.

GRAD
Dialysis Tub

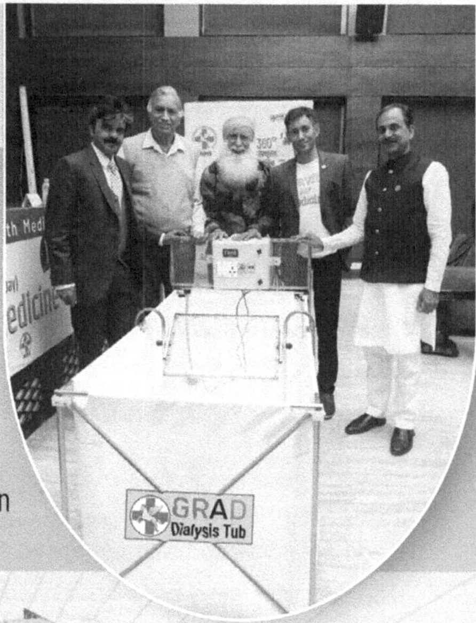

- Pain Management
- Cancer Therapy
- Self Dialysis
- Heart Attack prevention
- Curing Insomnia & Depression

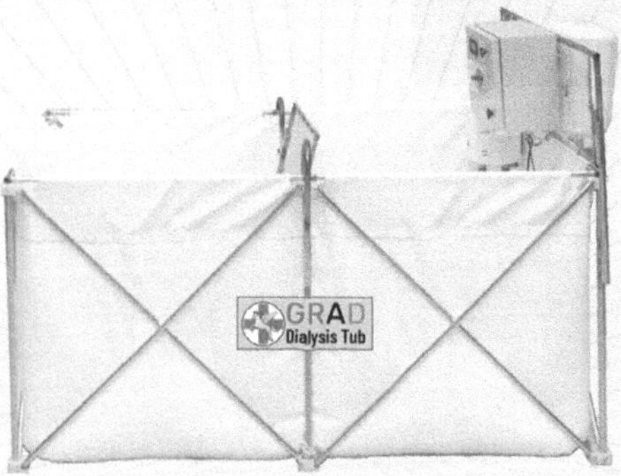

To design your own personal GRAD-Dialysis Tub

go to www.biswaroop.com/Dialysistub

The bath tub that cleanses your body from inside

Let every morning be the Hunza Morning

If you have decided to pick only one of my suggestions for the sake of your health, then take this suggestion:

Stop consuming tea specially, morning tea. The early morning tea makes the inner lining of your intestinal wall acidic, as after a long night of fasting your stomach is empty and craving for food. An acidic stomach on a regular basis is the single biggest cause of all kind of inflammatory and lifestyle diseases including arthritis, Diabetes etc.

How to stop craving of tea → Switch to Hunza Tea

Hunza Civilization: Hunza people are the Indians living at extreme northwest of India in Hindu Kush range. They are known to be one of the world's healthiest civilizations, often living up to the age of 110 years.

How to prepare Hunza Tea (serves four):

Ingredients:

- 12 Mint leaves(Pudina)
- 8 Basil Leaves(Tulsi)
- 4 Green cardamom (Elaichi)
- 2 gm Cinnamon (Dalchini)
- 20 gm Ginger (Adrak)
- 20 gm Jaggery (Gur)

Instructions:

- Take 4 cups of water in a tea pan
- Add all ingredients, simmer it for 10mins
- Add a dash of lemon juice and serve hot or cold